KEY TO OBESITY

"UNLOCKING THE SECRET AND REGAIN BODY SHAPE "

By Anthony J. Newton

Table of contents

Chapter 3
III. Health Consequences of Obesity
- Chronic diseases associated with obesity (diabetes, heart disease, etc.)
- Impact on mental health (depression, anxiety, etc.)
- Reduced quality of life

Chapter 4
IV. Weight Management Strategies
- Healthy eating habits (portion control, balanced diet, etc.)
- Physical activity recommendations
- Behavior change strategies (goal-setting, tracking progress, etc.)
- Role of healthcare professionals (nutritionists, physicians, etc.)

Chapter 5
V. Medical Interventions for Obesity
- Medications for weight loss

Chapter 8
VIII. Maintaining Long-Term Success
    - Strategies for maintaining weight loss and preventing weight regain
        - Setting realistic goals and monitoring progress
Overcoming setbacks and staying motivated

Chapter 9
IX. Conclusion
    - Importance of addressing obesity for overall health and well-being
        - Final thoughts and recommendations for managing obesity.

Chapter 1

Introduction

Obesity is a boundless worldwide issue that influences individuals from different backgrounds and age sections, representing a significant general wellbeing concern around the world. The World Wellbeing Association (WHO) describes corpulence as the amassing of excess muscle to fat ratio that jeopardizes wellbeing. This mind boggling and complex condition is impacted by a blend of hereditary, natural, and social elements, highlighting the significance of understanding its starting points and results in an all encompassing way.

Throughout the course of recent many years, there has been an exceptional and concerning expansion in corpulence rates, arriving at plague levels. Current insights from the World Wellbeing Association (WHO) show that north of 650 million grown-ups and 340 million kids and young people are presently sorted as overweight or corpulent. This quick acceleration features the prompt need for carrying out powerful techniques to handle this basic general medical problem.

Other than worries connected with appearance, stoutness has significant ramifications for wellbeing. It enormously elevates the gamble of creating persistent circumstances like sort 2 diabetes, coronary illness, stroke, and explicit kinds of malignant growth. Moreover, it adversely influences mental prosperity, confidence, connections, and by and large personal satisfaction.

The financial results of corpulence are huge, as medical services costs related with heftiness are projected to arrive at billions of dollars every year. Successfully tending to and forestalling heftiness requires an all encompassing methodology that thinks about numerous features of people's lives, including hereditary variables, ecological impacts, and standards of conduct.

Created by a regarded teacher with broad mastery in the field, this digital book expects to furnish perusers with a thorough outline of the causes and chance variables related with corpulence. It dives into the wellbeing results connected to stoutness and blueprints proof based systems for its powerful administration and avoidance. Additionally, the digital book reveals insight into the critical pretended by medical services experts in tending to weight and presents the most recent examination discoveries and arising patterns in the field.

Whether you are specifically managing corpulence or looking for preventive measures, this digital book furnishes you with fundamental data and apparatuses to come to informed conclusions about your wellbeing. By acquiring a more profound comprehension of the mind boggling nature of weight and investigating accessible administration methodologies, you can proactively assume command over your wellbeing and improve your general personal satisfaction. Together, let us leave on an excursion to battle heftiness and cultivate a better future for all.

Sarah's Change
This section follows the exceptional excursion of Sarah, a lady who confronted the difficulties of weight and went through an extraordinary change to recover her wellbeing and prosperity.

Sarah's battle with weight issues began right off the bat in her life. Restricted admittance to nutritious food choices and an absence of understanding about proper nutrition led to gradual weight gain. This affected her self-esteem and overall quality of life.

As she entered adulthood, Sarah found herself trapped in unhealthy eating habits and a sedentary lifestyle. Seeking comfort in sugary snacks and processed meals, she struggled to break free from this cycle. Concerned about her weight and the potential health risks it posed, Sarah's wake-up call came during a routine doctor's visit.

Determined to regain control over her life, Sarah embarked on a transformative journey towards better health. Recognizing the need for a comprehensive approach, she focused not only on her eating habits but also her mindset and physical activity levels.

Seeking guidance from healthcare professionals, Sarah consulted with a registered dietitian and a personal trainer. The dietitian helped her develop a personalized meal plan that emphasized balanced nutrition, portion control, and the inclusion of whole foods. Simultaneously, Sarah incorporated physical activity into her daily routine, starting with small steps and gradually progressing to more challenging workouts.

Though faced with obstacles and moments of doubt, Sarah remained committed to her goals. Support from online communities and local groups played a crucial role in her journey. Over time, she experienced significant positive changes, including increased energy levels, improved physical strength, and noticeable improvements in her overall well-being.

Sarah's transformation extended beyond the physical. She shifted her mindset, embracing self-care and self-love, understanding that her worth was not defined by her weight. Celebrating milestones along the way, Sarah began to appreciate her body and nourish it with wholesome foods that fueled her for a vibrant life.

Inspired by her own journey, Sarah became an advocate for healthy living and obesity awareness. Sharing her story through various platforms, she aimed to empower others facing similar challenges, providing them with support, knowledge, and inspiration to embark on their own transformative paths.

Sarah's story exemplifies the power of determination, resilience, and the capacity for change. Through her unwavering commitment to her health, she not only transformed her physical appearance but also gained a renewed sense of self-confidence and purpose. Her journey serves as an inspiration to countless individuals struggling with obesity, showing them that with the right mindset, support system, and lifestyle changes, they too can achieve lasting transformation and embrace a healthier, happier life.

Chapter 2

Causes and Risk Factors of Obesity

Genetic Factors

Hereditary qualities assumes a huge part in the improvement of weight. Studies have demonstrated the way that hereditary qualities can represent up to 70% of a singular's gamble of creating corpulence. Certain qualities can impact the digestion of fat, chemicals that control craving, and the stockpiling of fat in the body.

There are a few hereditary elements that have been connected to the improvement of heftiness, including:

Fat capacity and digestion qualities: A few qualities are liable for managing the manner in which the body stores and processes fat. Varieties in these qualities can influence a singular's capacity to consume calories, prompting weight gain and heftiness.

Craving controlling qualities: Chemicals, for example, leptin, ghrelin, and insulin direct craving and appetite signs. Hereditary varieties in these chemicals can prompt gorging and weight gain.

Energy consumption qualities: Energy use alludes to the quantity of calories a singular consumes while very still or during actual work. Varieties in qualities liable for energy consumption can prompt a more slow digestion, causing it harder to consume calories and get thinner.

While hereditary qualities assumes a critical part in the improvement of corpulence, it isn't the sole deciding variable. Ecological and conduct factors, for example, unfortunate dietary patterns and absence of active work, additionally add to weight gain and heftiness.

It's essential to take note of that regardless of whether an individual has a hereditary inclination to heftiness, solid way of life propensities can help forestall and deal with the condition. A mix of smart dieting propensities, ordinary actual work, and clinical administration can help people accomplish and keep a solid weight, no matter what their hereditary cosmetics.

Way of life Propensities

Way of life propensities are a significant supporter of the improvement of weight. Horrible eating routine, absence of actual work, and lacking rest can all prompt weight gain and corpulence.

1. Diet: A solid eating routine is fundamental for keeping a sound weight and forestalling stoutness. An eating regimen high in calories, unfortunate fats, and sugar can add to weight gain and stoutness. Handled food varieties, cheap food, and sweet drinks are normal guilty parties. An eating regimen ailing in natural products, vegetables, and incline

protein can likewise add to weight gain.

To keep a solid weight, it is critical to follow a decent eating routine that incorporates:

- Leafy foods: These give fundamental supplements, fiber, and cell reinforcements that assist with supporting in general wellbeing and forestall ongoing illnesses.

- Lean protein: Pick protein sources like lean meats, fish, eggs, vegetables, and nuts. These give fundamental amino acids expected to muscle development and fix.

- Entire grains: These give fiber, nutrients, and minerals that are fundamental for good wellbeing. Pick entire grain bread, pasta, rice, and oats.

- Sound fats: Pick sources like nuts, seeds, avocados, and greasy fish. These give fundamental unsaturated fats that are significant for heart wellbeing.

2. Actual work: Absence of actual work is one more key supporter of stoutness. A stationary way of life, described by delayed times of sitting or latency, can inability to burn calories and add to the collection of fat in the body. Normal active work, like energetic strolling, running, or strength preparing, can assist with supporting digestion, consume calories, and lessen the gamble of heftiness.

The American Heart Affiliation suggests no less than 150 minutes of moderate-power high-impact action or 75 minutes of energetic oxygen consuming movement each week for grown-ups. It is additionally essential to take part in muscle-reinforcing exercises somewhere around two times seven days.

3. Rest: Lacking rest can likewise add to weight gain and heftiness. Absence of rest can influence chemicals that manage hunger, prompting indulging and weight gain. Grown-ups ought to hold back nothing long stretches of rest each night to help by and large wellbeing and keep a sound weight.

In outline, way of life propensities assume a critical part in the improvement of weight. A solid eating routine, normal active work, and adequate rest are fundamental for keeping a sound weight and forestalling corpulence. By rolling out little improvements to your way of life propensities, you can work on your general wellbeing and diminish the gamble of corpulence.

C. Ailments

Certain ailments can add to weight gain and corpulence. These include:

1. Hypothyroidism: Hypothyroidism is a condition wherein the thyroid organ doesn't create an adequate number of chemicals. This can prompt weight

gain and trouble shedding pounds, as the thyroid chemicals assume a key part in directing digestion.

2. Cushing's disorder: Cushing's condition is an uncommon condition wherein the body creates an excess of cortisol, a chemical that directs digestion and the body's reaction to stretch. This can prompt weight gain, particularly in the chest area and face.

3. Polycystic ovary condition (PCOS): PCOS is a hormonal problem that influences ladies. It is portrayed by an awkwardness of chemicals, including insulin, which can prompt weight gain and trouble shedding pounds.

4. Prader-Willi condition: Prader-Willi condition is a hereditary problem that

influences craving guideline. Individuals with this condition frequently have a consistent sensation of yearning, which can prompt indulging and heftiness.

5. Rest apnea: Rest apnea is a condition where an individual's breathing is intruded on during rest. This can prompt unfortunate rest quality, exhaustion, and weight gain.

6. Other ailments: Other ailments, like insulin obstruction, type 2 diabetes, and certain meds, can likewise add to weight gain and heftiness.

On the off chance that you have any of these ailments, it means quite a bit to work with your medical services supplier to oversee them and limit their effect on your weight. Now and again, clinical treatment might be important to deal with these circumstances and forestall further weight gain.

D. Financial Variables:
Financial variables can assume a critical part in the improvement of weight. These variables can include:

1. Pay: Low pay can restrict admittance to quality food sources and safe spots to work out, making it more challenging to keep a solid weight.

2. Schooling: Lower levels of instruction can be related with lower wellbeing education, making it harder for people to settle on sound decisions

and grasp the results of undesirable ways of behaving.

3. Climate: The fabricated climate, including admittance to supermarkets, walkways, and safe parks, can affect a singular's capacity to take part in sound ways of behaving.

4. Culture: Social mentalities and convictions about body weight and food can influence a singular's dietary patterns and actual work levels.

5. Stress: Ongoing pressure, frequently connected with low financial status, can build the gamble of corpulence by setting off the arrival of chemicals that advance weight gain.

6. Separation: Segregation in view of race, identity, or different variables can prompt constant pressure, restricted open doors, and decreased admittance to assets that advance sound ways of behaving.

It means a lot to address these financial variables in endeavors to forestall and treat weight. Approaches and projects that elevate admittance to good food varieties, safe spots to work out, and different assets can assist with tending to these abberations and advance better ways of behaving. Moreover, expanding mindfulness and comprehension of the effect of these elements on wellbeing can assist with diminishing shame and advance sympathy and backing for people and networks impacted by heftiness.

Section 1: Causes and Risk Factors

- Genetic factors: Explore how Sarah's family history of obesity influenced her weight gain, highlighting the role of genetics in her obesity.

- Lifestyle habits: Discuss Sarah's upbringing in a household with unhealthy eating patterns and limited physical activity, emphasizing the impact of these habits on her weight.

- Environmental factors: Examine the influence of Sarah's surroundings, including easy access to processed foods and sedentary lifestyles, on her obesity.

- Psychological factors: Analyze Sarah's emotional relationship with food, including stress, emotional eating, and other psychological factors that contributed to her weight gain.

- Socioeconomic factors: Highlight the impact of socioeconomic factors such as limited access to nutritious food and healthcare disparities on Sarah's ability to maintain a healthy weight.

Section 2: Sarah's Struggles with Obesity
- Childhood experiences: Share personal anecdotes about Sarah's early experiences with weight gain, including the challenges she faced at school and the impact on her self-esteem.
- Adolescent years: Discuss how societal pressures, body image issues, and peer influence affected Sarah's relationship with her body and contributed to her struggle with obesity during her teenage years.

- Adulthood challenges: Explore the various challenges Sarah faced as an adult, such as work-related stress, time constraints,
and the difficulties of managing her weight while juggling multiple responsibilities.

Section 3: Seeking Help and Support
- Self-reflection and realization: Detail the moment Sarah realized the need to address her obesity and make positive changes in her life.
- Professional guidance: Discuss Sarah's journey to find healthcare professionals, nutritionists, and personal trainers who provided expert guidance and support in her weight loss journey.

- Emotional support: Highlight the importance of Sarah's network of family, friends, and support groups in providing emotional support, motivation, and accountability throughout her weight loss journey.

Section 4: Overcoming Obstacles and Achieving Success
- Sarah's strategies and lifestyle changes: Explore the specific strategies and lifestyle modifications Sarah implemented to achieve her weight loss goals, including dietary changes, regular physical activity, and stress management techniques.
- Celebrating milestones: Share the significant milestones Sarah achieved along her journey, such as reaching specific weight loss targets, improving

health markers, and gaining confidence and self-esteem.
- Maintaining long-term success: Discuss the challenges of weight maintenance and the strategies Sarah adopted to sustain her healthy lifestyle and prevent weight regain.

By delving into Sarah's experiences with the various factors contributing to her obesity, you be able to gain a comprehensive understanding of the complexities involved in weight gain and the obstacles faced by individuals on similar journeys. Sarah's story serves as an relatable and inspiring narrative, offering insights, guidance, and motivation for you seeking to overcome obesity and achieve lasting health and well-being.

Chapter 3

Health Consequences of Obesity

Corpulence can adversely affect wellbeing, including:

1. Cardiovascular illness: Stoutness is a significant gamble factor for cardiovascular sickness, including hypertension, coronary illness, and stroke.

2. Type 2 diabetes: Weight builds the gamble of creating type 2 diabetes, a constant condition in which the body can't as expected use and store glucose (sugar).

3. Disease: Weight has been connected to an expanded gamble of a few kinds

of malignant growth, including bosom, colon, and pancreatic disease.

4. Respiratory issues: Weight can make it harder to inhale and expand the gamble of conditions like rest apnea, asthma, and persistent obstructive pneumonic illness (COPD).

5. Joint issues: Overabundance weight can overwhelm the joints, prompting conditions like osteoarthritis.

6. Psychological wellness: Weight has been connected to an expanded gamble of sadness, uneasiness, and other emotional well-being conditions.

7. Regenerative wellbeing: Weight can influence conceptive wellbeing in all kinds of people, prompting issues like

fruitlessness and entanglements during pregnancy.

8. Abbreviated life expectancy: Corpulence is related with a more limited life expectancy, with research recommending that it can diminish future by quite a long while.

It means quite a bit to address weight to forestall or moderate these negative wellbeing outcomes. This can include making way of life changes like further developing eating routine and expanding active work, as well as looking for clinical treatment or backing from a medical services supplier. By tending to corpulence, people can work on their general wellbeing and personal satisfaction.

Sarah's Struggles with Obesity-Related Consequences

Section 1: Health Consequences

- Physical health challenges: Explore the various health issues that Sarah encountered as a result of her obesity, such as high blood pressure, diabetes, joint pain, and sleep apnea. Emphasize the profound impact of these conditions on her overall well-being and quality of life, drawing upon scientific evidence that links obesity to these health problems.

- Mental and emotional toll: Discuss the psychological effects of obesity on Sarah, including feelings of low self-esteem, depression, and anxiety. Explain the underlying mechanisms that contribute to these mental health struggles in individuals with obesity, referencing research findings from psychology and psychiatry.

- Social implications: Address the impact of obesity on Sarah's social life, including experiences of isolation, discrimination, and limited participation in certain activities due to physical limitations. Discuss the societal factors that contribute to the stigmatization of obesity and the importance of fostering a more inclusive and understanding environment.

Section 2: Failed Attempts and Setbacks

- Yo-yo dieting: Detail Sarah's experiences with various fad diets and weight loss programs that she attempted but ultimately couldn't sustain. Explain the physiological and psychological factors that make long-term weight loss challenging and the potential negative consequences of repeated weight cycling.

- Emotional eating and binge episodes: Explore how Sarah used food as a coping mechanism for emotional stress and occasionally engaged in episodes of binge eating, hindering her progress in managing her health. Discuss the interplay between emotions, stress, and eating behaviors, referencing research in the fields of psychology and behavioral science.

- Lack of support and understanding: Discuss the challenges Sarah faced in receiving adequate support from healthcare professionals, friends, and family members who may have underestimated the severity of her struggles or dismissed her efforts to make positive changes. Highlight the importance of a multidisciplinary approach and empathetic care in addressing obesity-related challenges.

Section 3: Overcoming Challenges and Seeking Solutions
- Mindset shift: Highlight the pivotal moment when Sarah decided to take control of her health and adopted a new mindset focused on self-compassion, determination, and long-term well-being. Discuss the psychological principles and techniques that can facilitate mindset shifts and promote sustainable behavior change.
- Seeking professional help: Discuss Sarah's journey in finding a supportive healthcare team, including doctors, nutritionists, and therapists, who

provided guidance and personalized strategies to address her specific challenges. Emphasize the role of evidence-based interventions, such as cognitive-behavioral therapy and lifestyle counseling, in supporting individuals with obesity.

- Building a support network: Address the importance of surrounding oneself with a supportive community, whether through support groups, online forums, or understanding friends and family members. Discuss the potential benefits of social support in promoting behavior change and maintaining long-term success.

Section 4: Triumph and Growth
- Small victories and progress: Share the milestones and achievements Sarah experienced along her journey,

such as significant weight loss, improvements in health markers, and increased energy and vitality. Highlight the scientific evidence on the positive effects of weight loss on health outcomes and the potential for sustainable lifestyle changes.

- Lessons learned: Discuss the valuable insights Sarah gained through her struggles, such as the significance of self-care, self-acceptance, and perseverance. Explore how these lessons align with scientific principles of behavior change and reference relevant studies and theories.

- Inspiring others: Highlight Sarah's desire to share her story and inspire others facing similar challenges, motivating them to embark on their own health journeys and overcome obstacles. Discuss the importance of narratives and personal experiences in public health communication and the potential for peer support in fostering positive health behaviors.

By illuminating Sarah's struggles and challenges in managing her health due to obesity-related consequences, readers gain a deeper understanding of the complexities involved in overcoming these difficulties.

Chapter 4

Weight Management Strategie

Weight the board procedures can help people accomplish and keep a sound weight, decreasing the gamble of heftiness and related medical issues. A few powerful methodologies include:

1. Solid eating routine: Eating an eating routine wealthy in natural products, vegetables, entire grains, and incline proteins can assist people with keeping a sound weight and decrease the gamble of constant illnesses.

2. Actual work: Ordinary actual work can assist people with consuming calories and keep a sound weight, while likewise working on by and large wellbeing and prosperity.

3. Changing outwardly: Working on propensities and ways of behaving around eating, work out, and other way of life variables can assist people with rolling out manageable improvements and keep a solid load over the long run.

4. Medicine: Certain meds, for example, weight reduction medications or meds for related conditions like diabetes, can assist people with dealing with their weight.

5. Medical procedure: now and again, weight reduction medical procedure might be suggested for people with extreme stoutness who have not had the option to accomplish weight reduction through different strategies.

It is essential to take note of that weight the board techniques ought to be individualized and custom-made to every individual's special necessities and conditions. Talking with a medical services supplier or enrolled dietitian can assist people with fostering a successful weight the executives plan that is protected and maintainable. By embracing sound propensities and looking for proper clinical help, people can accomplish and keep a solid weight, decreasing the gamble of stoutness and related medical conditions.

Sarah's Path to Embracing Healthier Lifestyle Practices and Overcoming Hurdles

Section 1: The Decision to Change
- Reflective contemplation: Sarah engages in introspection, examining her previous endeavors to adopt healthier lifestyle practices and the obstacles she encountered. She acknowledges recurring patterns of self-sabotage and impediments that impeded her progress.
- A transformative moment: Sarah experiences a transformative event that catalyzes her motivation to effect lasting change. Whether it stems from a health scare, personal epiphany, or a

paradigm shift in her perspective, she discerns the imperative of prioritizing her well-being and commits to embracing healthier habits.

- Goal formulation: Sarah establishes well-defined and attainable objectives across various dimensions of her life, encompassing weight management, physical fitness, mental wellness, and overall health enhancement. She recognizes the significance of setting Specific, Measurable, Achievable, Relevant, and Time-bound (SMART) goals.

Section 2: Overcoming Adversities

- Identifying individual challenges: Sarah recognizes the unique challenges she faces on her journey to adopt healthier habits. These obstacles may encompass emotional eating, sedentary lifestyle tendencies, time constraints for meal preparation or exercise, and limited access to resources or support systems.

- Devising strategies for success: Sarah explores diverse strategies to surmount her impediments and sustain commitment to her goals. She acquaints herself with techniques for managing emotional eating, innovatively incorporates physical activity into her daily routine, and proactively seeks out resources and support networks to overcome the barriers encountered.

- Cultivating resilience: Sarah internalizes the understanding that setbacks are inherent to transformative journeys. She learns to rebound from setbacks, leveraging them as opportunities for growth and knowledge acquisition. Sarah develops resilience and an optimistic mindset, enabling her to persevere through challenging circumstances.

Section 3: Embracing Healthier Lifestyle Practices
- Nutrition and meal planning: Sarah engages in self-education regarding nutrition, acquiring knowledge to make informed food choices and cultivate balanced meal plans. She grasps the importance of portion control, mindful eating, and integration of nutrient-rich foods into her diet. Sarah experiments with novel recipes and explores diverse culinary techniques to imbue healthy eating with pleasure and sustainability.

- Regular physical activity: Sarah integrates regular physical activity into her daily regimen. She explores various exercise modalities such as walking, jogging, strength training, yoga, or dance, aiming to discover activities that provide both enjoyment and fitness benefits. Sarah establishes realistic exercise goals and progressively enhances her fitness levels, bolstering strength and endurance.

- Stress management and self-care: Sarah imbibes the significance of stress management and self-care in maintaining a wholesome lifestyle. She embraces practices like meditation, deep breathing exercises, journaling, and engagement in activities that foster joy and relaxation. Sarah elevates the priority of her mental and

emotional well-being, understanding that self-care is instrumental in fostering overall health.
- Seeking expert guidance: Sarah acknowledges the value of seeking professional guidance and support. She consults with healthcare professionals such as physicians, registered dietitians, and therapists, who offer tailored recommendations and evidence-based strategies to address specific challenges. Sarah actively participates in workshops, classes, or support groups tailored to her needs, augmenting her guidance and motivation.

Section 4: Celebrating Progress and Sustaining Achievements
- Milestones and accomplishments: Sarah celebrates her milestones and

achievements along the trajectory. She acknowledges and rewards herself for attaining various milestones, be it weight loss, improved fitness levels, augmented energy levels, enhanced sleep patterns, or overall health advancements.

- Lifestyle as an ongoing journey: Sarah embraces the understanding that adopting healthier lifestyle practices constitutes an ongoing journey rather than a quick fix. She espouses the mindset that progress, rather than perfection, is key. Sarah remains steadfast in.

Chapter 5

Medical Interventions for Obesity

Notwithstanding way of life changes, clinical intercessions might be fundamental for certain people with heftiness. These intercessions can include:

1. Meds: Physician endorsed prescriptions, for example, craving suppressants or weight reduction medications might be suggested for people with corpulence who have not had the option to accomplish weight reduction through way of life changes alone.

2. Bariatric medical procedure: Otherwise called weight reduction medical procedure, bariatric medical procedure can assist people with serious corpulence accomplish critical weight reduction by changing the stomach related framework.

3. Clinical weight the executives programs: These projects include an extensive way to deal with weight the board, including clinical management, diet and exercise guiding, and other help administrations.

It is vital to take note of that clinical intercessions for weight ought to be painstakingly thought of and individualized to every individual's remarkable necessities and conditions. Talking with a medical care supplier or weight reduction expert can assist people with deciding whether clinical mediations are proper and which choices might be best for them.Sarah's decision-making process and her experiences with medical interventions were essential components of her journey towards improved health and well-being. Let's explore the details of how Sarah made her decisions and the different medical interventions she tried.

1. Assessing Health Needs and Goals:
Sarah started by evaluating her health needs and setting clear goals. She identified areas of concern like weight management, physical fitness, and overall well-being. This assessment helped Sarah establish a foundation for making informed decisions.

2. Researching Medical Interventions:
Sarah conducted extensive research to gather information about available medical interventions. She consulted reliable sources, including healthcare professionals, scientific literature, and online resources. This research allowed her to understand the range of interventions and their potential benefits and risks.

3. Consulting with Healthcare Professionals:
Recognizing the importance of professional guidance, Sarah sought the expertise of healthcare professionals. She consulted doctors, nutritionists, and specialists who provided valuable insights into her health conditions and recommended

suitable interventions. These consultations helped Sarah gain a better understanding of her options and ensured that her decisions were based on expert advice.

4. Weighing Benefits and Risks:
Sarah carefully considered the potential benefits and risks associated with each intervention. She evaluated factors such as effectiveness, potential side effects, long-term outcomes, and impact on her quality of life. This careful assessment allowed her to make informed decisions and prioritize interventions that aligned with her goals and values.

5. Lifestyle Changes:

Sarah acknowledged the importance of making lifestyle modifications to achieve her health goals. She embraced changes in her diet, exercise routine, sleep habits, and stress management techniques. Despite the challenges, Sarah remained committed to these adjustments, as she observed positive changes in her overall health and well-being.

6. Medication:
In certain cases, Sarah was advised to take medication as part of her intervention plan. She diligently followed the prescribed medications, paying attention to potential side effects and effectiveness. Sarah maintained open communication with her healthcare providers, reporting any concerns or changes in her

condition. Through this process, she gained a deeper understanding of how medications played a role in managing her health.

7. Surgical Interventions:
For specific health conditions, Sarah considered surgical interventions such as bariatric surgery or weight loss procedures. She extensively researched these options, sought expert advice, and evaluated the potential risks and benefits. Sarah underwent a thorough preoperative proccss and proceeded with the surgical procedure. Afterward, she made necessary lifestyle adjustments to ensure the long-term success of the interventions. The surgical interventions had a positive impact on

her weight management and overall health, contributing to her well-being.

8. Complementary and Alternative Therapies:

Sarah explored complementary and alternative therapies to enhance her health journey. These included practices such as acupuncture, herbal medicine, and mindfulness techniques. While some interventions provided additional benefits and support, Sarah was mindful of relying on evidence-based approaches and consulted with healthcare professionals to ensure their safety and effectiveness.

9. Evaluating Results and Adjustments:

Throughout her journey, Sarah regularly assessed the results of each intervention. She monitored her progress, noting both positive outcomes and any challenges encountered. Based on these evaluations, Sarah made adjustments to her treatment plans when necessary, ensuring that her interventions remained aligned with her evolving health needs and goals.

Sarah's decision-making process and experiences with medical interventions demonstrate her commitment to achieving optimal health. By conducting thorough research, seeking professional advice, and carefully considering the benefits and risks, Sarah empowered herself to make informed decisions and customize her interventions according to her specific requirements. Through this journey, Sarah gained valuable insights, resilience, and a renewed sense of well-being.

Chapter 6

Psychological and Emotional Factors

Corpulence can have huge mental and close to home effects, which can thusly influence weight the executives endeavors. A few normal mental and profound variables related with heftiness include:

1. Stress: Constant pressure can prompt indulging and weight gain, and can put forth weight the board attempts more troublesome.

2. Sorrow and tension: People with stoutness are at higher gamble for

wretchedness and nervousness, which can thusly influence dietary patterns and weight the executives.

3.   Self-perception: Negative self-perception and low confidence can make it hard for people with stoutness to make supportable way of life changes and keep a solid weight.

4. Food compulsion: A few people with stoutness might battle with food enslavement, making it hard to control dietary patterns and accomplish weight reduction.

Tending to mental and close to home variables is a significant part of weight the board and by and large wellbeing. A few systems for tending to these elements include:

1.   Treatment: Working with a specialist or guide can assist people with resolving basic close to home and mental issues connected with stoutness and foster successful survival techniques.

Sarah's health journey encompassed not only physical challenges but also emotional struggles that she had to confront and overcome. Let's explore Sarah's emotional struggles and the steps she took to conquer them:

1. Self-Doubt and Low Self-Esteem:
Sarah often grappled with self-doubt and low self-esteem, particularly regarding her body image and weight. She frequently compared herself to societal ideals, which left her feeling

inadequate. To surmount these emotional obstacles, Sarah sought guidance from a therapist who aided her in cultivating a positive self-image and nurturing self-compassion. Through therapy, she learned to value herself beyond physical appearance and embrace her unique qualities.

2. Fear of Failure and Persistent Setbacks:
Sarah encountered moments of fear and discouragement, especially when faced with setbacks in her health journey. She harbored concerns about not achieving her goals and worried that her efforts would be futile. To conquer these emotional barriers, Sarah adopted a growth mindset. She acknowledged that setbacks were an integral part of the process and viewed

them as valuable opportunities for growth. Sarah exhibited resilience and perseverance, staying motivated despite the challenges she encountered.

3. Emotional Eating and Coping Mechanisms:

Sarah relied on food as a coping mechanism to deal with her emotions, often resorting to emotional eating during times of stress or difficulty. Recognizing that this unhealthy habit hindered her progress and emotional well-being, Sarah sought assistance from a nutritionist who guided her in developing healthier coping strategies. Through therapy and guidance, she acquired alternative ways to manage her emotions, such as engaging in physical activity, practicing mindfulness, and seeking support from others.

4. Overcoming Shame and Seeking Support:
Sarah grappled with feelings of shame and embarrassment regarding her weight struggles, making it challenging for her to seek support from others. However, she gradually opened up to trusted friends and family members who formed a strong support network. Sarah discovered the power of vulnerability and realized that she was not alone on her journey. By sharing her challenges and receiving support, she found strength and encouragement to continue moving forward.

5. Celebrating Non-Scale Victories:
Sarah recognized the significance of celebrating victories that extended beyond mere numbers on the scale. Rather than solely focusing on weight loss, she celebrated achievements such as increased energy levels, improved physical fitness, better sleep patterns, and enhanced mental well-being. By shifting her attention to these non-scale victories, Sarah nurtured a more positive mindset and acknowledged her progress beyond the confines of weight alone.

6. Building a Supportive Community:
Sarah proactively sought out a community of individuals who shared similar health goals and faced similar challenges. She joined support groups, online communities, and fitness

classes where she encountered like-minded individuals who provided encouragement and shared their own experiences. Being part of a supportive community allowed Sarah to feel understood, motivated, and less isolated in her struggles.

7. Cultivating Mindfulness and Emotional Awareness:
Sarah incorporated mindfulness practices into her daily life to develop emotional awareness and regulate her responses to stress and negative emotions. Through meditation, deep breathing exercises, and mindfulness techniques, she honed her ability to recognize and navigate her emotions in a healthy and balanced manner. This heightened self-awareness empowered Sarah to manage her

emotional struggles more effectively and make conscious choices that supported her overall well-being.

By confronting her emotional struggles head-on, Sarah took significant strides toward conquering them. Through therapy, self-reflection, seeking support, and practicing mindfulness, she fostered resilience, self-compassion, and a more positive outlook. Sarah's emotional transformation played a pivotal role in her health journey, equipping her with the strength and determination to navigate challenges with confidence.

2. Mindfulness practices: Mindfulness practices such as meditation or yoga can help individuals manage stress and improve emotional well-being.

3. Support groups: Participating in support groups or other group therapy can provide individuals with social support and a sense of community, which can be helpful for addressing emotional and psychological factors related to obesity.

By addressing psychological and emotional factors alongside lifestyle changes and medical interventions, individuals can achieve sustainable weight loss and improve overall health and well-being.

Chapter 7

Childhood Obesity

Youth weight is a developing worry, with paces of young life stoutness expanding fundamentally throughout recent many years. Youth stoutness can fundamentally affect wellbeing, both in adolescence and sometime down the road. A portion of the wellbeing results of young life weight include:

1. Expanded hazard of constant sicknesses: Youngsters who are fat are at expanded risk for creating persistent infections like sort 2

diabetes, coronary illness, and certain malignant growths.

2. Mental effects: Adolescence stoutness can likewise have mental effects, including expanded chance of discouragement, nervousness, and low confidence.

3. Social effects: Youngsters who are fat may likewise encounter social disgrace and segregation, which can additionally influence their mental prosperity.

Factors adding to adolescence heftiness include:

1. Diet: Unfortunate dietary decisions, for example, polishing off high measures of handled food varieties

and sweet beverages, can add to adolescence weight.

2. Actual work: Absence of active work and inactive ways of behaving, for example, exorbitant screen time, can likewise add to youth weight.

3. Hereditary qualities: Hereditary qualities can assume a part in youth corpulence, with offspring of large guardians being at higher gamble.

Tending to youth heftiness requires a complete methodology that includes both the singular kid and their loved ones. Techniques for tending to youth corpulence include:

1. Smart dieting: Empowering kids to consume a solid and adjusted diet can

help forestall and oversee youth heftiness.

2. Actual work: Empowering kids to participate in normal active work, like playing sports or partaking in dynamic play, can help forestall and oversee adolescence heftiness.

3. Family contribution: Including the entire family in endeavors to forestall and oversee youth stoutness can assist with establishing a strong and sound climate for the kid.

By tending to youth heftiness from the beginning, people can diminish their gamble of persistent sicknesses and work on their general wellbeing and prosperity all through their lives.

Sarah's childhood obesity had a significant impact on her life, affecting her physical, emotional, and social well-being. Let's explore Sarah's journey, including the challenges she faced and the lasting effects of childhood obesity:

1. Early Signs and Challenges:

From a young age, Sarah struggled with weight-related issues that affected her overall health and well-being. She encountered difficulties managing her weight, experiencing excessive weight gain as a persistent concern. Sarah's physical abilities were limited, making it challenging for her to participate in regular exercise and activities like her peers.

2. Emotional and Psychological Impact:
Childhood obesity took a toll on Sarah's emotional and psychological state. She experienced self-consciousness, low self-esteem, and social isolation due to the stigma associated with being overweight. Sarah faced bullying and teasing from her peers, intensifying her emotional struggles. Societal beauty standards and media representations further contributed to negative body image and emotional distress.

3. Health Consequences and Medical Conditions:

Sarah's childhood obesity put her at a higher risk of developing various health conditions. She faced an increased likelihood of chronic diseases such as type 2 diabetes, cardiovascular problems, and joint-related issues. Managing her blood pressure, cholesterol levels, and overall metabolic health presented challenges. The long-term health consequences emphasized the importance of early intervention and effective management.

4. Impact on Social Life and Relationships:
Childhood obesity affected Sarah's social life and relationships significantly. She often felt excluded from social activities due to her weight, leading to feelings of

loneliness and isolation. Sarah struggled to form friendships and establish a sense of belonging. The impact on her social interactions extended beyond childhood, leaving a lasting impact on her social development and well-being.

5. Academic Performance and Educational Challenges:
Sarah's childhood obesity also influenced her academic performance and educational experiences. Concentration, focus, and energy levels were affected, hindering her ability to fully engage in learning. Weight-related concerns impacted her self-confidence and academic progress. Overcoming these challenges required additional support and

understanding from educators and parents.

6. Family Dynamics and Support:
Sarah's family dynamics and support system were also affected by childhood obesity. Her parents and caregivers faced the challenge of addressing her weight-related concerns while creating a nurturing environment. Family support played a crucial role in providing emotional support, guidance, and access to resources for Sarah's journey towards improved health.

Sarah's childhood obesity left a lasting impact on her life. The physical, emotional, and social challenges she encountered shaped her perceptions, self-esteem, and overall quality of life.

However, Sarah's story is not defined solely by these challenges. Her journey highlights resilience, determination, and personal growth. Sharing her experiences, Sarah aims to inspire others facing similar struggles and advocate for greater awareness, support, and early intervention to address childhood obesity effectively.

Chapter 8

Maintaining Long-Term Success

Sustaining long-term success in weight management involves a holistic approach that encompasses strategies for maintaining weight loss, preventing weight regain, setting realistic goals, monitoring progress, overcoming setbacks, and staying motivated.

1. Strategies for Maintaining Weight Loss and Preventing Weight Regain:

To preserve weight loss and prevent regaining weight, it is important to incorporate various strategies:

- Regular Physical Activity: Engaging in consistent physical activity, including cardiovascular exercises, strength training, and flexibility exercises, helps maintain muscle mass, boost metabolism, and promote overall well-being.

- Balanced and Nutritious Diet: Following a well-rounded, nutritious diet that emphasizes whole foods like fruits, vegetables, lean proteins, whole grains, and healthy fats while limiting processed foods, sugary beverages, and high-calorie snacks supports weight maintenance and overall health.

- Portion Control: Practicing portion control by being mindful of serving sizes, using smaller plates, and listening to hunger and fullness cues prevents overeating and fosters healthy eating habits.

- Mindful Eating Habits: Adopting mindful eating habits, such as being present during meals, savoring each bite, and eating with awareness, cultivates a positive relationship with food, enhances satisfaction, and reduces mindless eating.

- Supportive Environment: Surrounding oneself with a supportive environment, including family, friends, or a weight loss community, provides encouragement, accountability, and understanding during the weight management journey.

- Regular Monitoring and Reflection: Monitoring progress through tools like food diaries, physical activity tracking, and regular weigh-ins facilitates self-reflection, identifies areas for adjustment, and helps maintain focus on long-term goals.

2. Setting Realistic Goals and Monitoring Progress:

Setting achievable goals that align with overall health and well-being is essential for long-term success. Breaking larger goals into smaller milestones and regularly monitoring progress through objective measures like weight, body measurements, and body composition analysis ensures accountability and identifies areas for improvement.

3. Overcoming Setbacks:

Approaching setbacks as learning opportunities and maintaining resilience are crucial in the weight management journey. Identifying triggers, seeking support from healthcare professionals or support groups, reevaluating strategies, and staying committed to long-term goals help overcome setbacks and maintain motivation. Embracing a growth mindset and focusing on progress rather than perfection are key principles.

4. Staying Motivated:

Sustaining motivation is vital for long-term success. Strategies for staying motivated include:

- Building a Support Network: Creating a supportive network of friends, family, or a weight loss community provides encouragement, understanding, and accountability. Sharing experiences, challenges, and successes with others on a similar path fosters motivation and offers valuable insights.

- Positive Self-Talk and Visualization: Engaging in positive self-talk and visualization techniques reinforces motivation and cultivates a positive mindset. Affirming one's capabilities and visualizing success can help maintain enthusiasm and determination.

By implementing these strategies and staying committed to long-term goals, individuals can maintain weight loss, prevent weight regain, and experience sustained success in their weight management journey

Sarah's ongoing journey to maintain her weight loss and lead a healthier life is a complex and dynamic process that requires unwavering dedication, consistent effort, and a holistic approach. After achieving her initial weight loss goals, Sarah understands the crucial importance of preserving her progress and ensuring sustainable success. She embraces various strategies and practices to sustain her weight loss and cultivate a healthier lifestyle, including:

1. Continuously Prioritizing Healthy Eating Habits:
Sarah recognizes the fundamental role of maintaining a balanced and nutritious diet in preserving her weight loss. She continues to prioritize the consumption of whole, unprocessed foods that are rich in essential nutrients such as fruits, vegetables, lean proteins, and whole grains. By practicing portion control, mindful eating, and following a well-rounded meal plan, Sarah establishes enduring healthy eating habits that support her long-term objectives.

2. Engaging in Regular Physical Activity:
Physical activity remains a cornerstone of Sarah's daily routine. She incorporates a diverse range of exercises including cardiovascular workouts, strength training, and flexibility exercises. By consistently engaging in physical activity, Sarah not only manages her weight effectively but also enjoys the numerous benefits of exercise such as improved cardiovascular health, increased energy levels, enhanced strength, and an overall sense of well-being.

3. Maintaining Self-Monitoring and Accountability:
Sarah understands the importance of ongoing self-monitoring to stay accountable and track her progress.

She diligently keeps a food journal, recording her meals, snacks, and beverages to heighten her awareness of her dietary patterns. Additionally, Sarah regularly monitors her weight, body measurements, and fitness achievements to accurately assess her progress and make any necessary adjustments to her routine.

4. Nurturing Emotional Well-being:
Sarah acknowledges that emotional well-being plays a vital role in sustaining weight loss. She places significant emphasis on self-care activities such as mindfulness practices, stress management techniques, and seeking support from her social network, including close friends, family members, or participation in support groups. By

actively addressing emotional triggers and developing healthy coping mechanisms, Sarah cultivates a positive mindset and emotional resilience that supports her long-term success.

5. Setting Realistic Long-Term Goals: Sarah proactively sets realistic and achievable long-term goals to maintain focus and motivation throughout her journey. She identifies specific targets aligned with her health and fitness aspirations, whether it's completing a charity run, mastering a new fitness skill, or achieving a certain body composition. Sarah breaks down these larger goals into smaller, manageable milestones, celebrating each achievement along the way, which

fuels her motivation and boosts her confidence.

6. Continuous Education and Self-Improvement:
Sarah is committed to expanding her knowledge about nutrition, exercise science, and overall well-being. She stays updated with the latest research findings, consults with healthcare professionals for expert guidance, and actively seeks opportunities to attend seminars, workshops, or educational programs that provide insights into sustainable weight management strategies. By actively pursuing continuous learning and staying informed, Sarah empowers herself to make well-informed decisions and adapt her lifestyle practices as needed.

7. Acknowledging and Celebrating Non-Scale Victories:
Sarah understands that success goes beyond the number on the scale. She wholeheartedly recognizes and celebrates non-scale victories that reflect positive changes in her life, such as increased energy levels, improved sleep quality, enhanced self-confidence, and an overall improved quality of life. By shifting her focus to these meaningful achievements, Sarah sustains her motivation and remains committed to long-tcrm health and well-being.

Through the consistent application of these strategies and her unwavering commitment to her health and well-being, Sarah embarks on an ongoing journey to maintain her weight loss and cultivate a healthier life. She acknowledges that long-term success requires a comprehensive approach that encompasses various aspects of her lifestyle, and she remains dedicated to making sustainable choices that support her overall health and vitality.

Chapter 9

Conclusion

Stoutness is a mind boggling and complex issue that influences a huge number of individuals all over the planet. Characterized as having overabundance muscle to fat ratio, weight is impacted by various variables including hereditary qualities, way of life propensities, and financial status. Heftiness has been connected to a scope of medical conditions, including persistent illnesses like sort 2 diabetes, coronary illness, and specific kinds of disease. It can likewise altogether affect mental prosperity, including expanded chance of sorrow, uneasiness, and low confidence.

Luckily, there are numerous procedures for forestalling and overseeing stoutness. Way of life changes, like eating a sound eating routine, expanding actual work, and getting sufficient rest, can all assist with decreasing the gamble of weight. Moreover, clinical mediations and weight the board procedures, for example, medicine and medical procedure can be compelling in aiding people accomplish and keep a solid weight.

Tending to stoutness requires a thorough methodology that includes people, families, medical care suppliers, and policymakers. On a singular level, it is essential to settle on sound decisions and way of life changes that advance a solid weight. This can incorporate looking for help from medical services suppliers, joining support gatherings, and making changes to one's eating regimen and work-out daily schedule. On a cultural level, essential to establish a climate upholds solid decisions, for example, carrying out strategies that advance good food choices, further developing admittance to active work, and lessening financial variations.

Sarah's remarkable transformation journey has been a profound testament to her unwavering commitment to her health and well-being. Throughout her path, she encountered numerous challenges and celebrated numerous victories, offering valuable lessons for those seeking a healthier and happier life.

One of the most significant lessons Sarah learned was the power of self-belief and empowerment. She discovered that having faith in herself and her ability to make positive changes enabled her to overcome any obstacle. Sarah's journey serves as a powerful example of how self-belief can empower individuals to take control of their health and make necessary lifestyle adjustments.

Another crucial lesson Sarah learned was the importance of patience and perseverance. She recognized that sustainable changes take time and setbacks are a natural part of the process. Instead of being discouraged by setbacks, Sarah embraced them as opportunities for growth and learning. Her unwavering determination and resilience enabled her to stay committed to her journey despite challenges.

Sarah also gained insights into the significance of a holistic approach to health and well-being. She realized that true transformation encompasses not only physical health but also mental and emotional well-being. Sarah embarked on a journey of self-discovery, practicing self-care, and seeking support from loved ones. By prioritizing her emotional health and developing a balanced mindset, she found herself better equipped to navigate challenges and maintain her overall well-being.

Setting realistic goals and celebrating milestones became essential components of Sarah's transformation journey. She understood that progress should be measured beyond the numbers on a scale. Improved energy levels, increased self-confidence, and enhanced well-being became markers of her success. Recognizing and celebrating these non-scale victories provided Sarah with the motivation and momentum to continue her journey.

Above all, Sarah's most profound lesson was the transformative power of self-love and self-acceptance. By embracing her body and recognizing her inherent worth beyond appearance, she experienced a profound shift in her relationship with herself. Sarah learned to treat herself with kindness, compassion, and respect, fostering a positive body image and a deep sense of self-worth. This newfound self-love became the foundation for her ongoing growth and transformation.

In summary, Sarah's transformation journey serves as an inspiration, demonstrating the strength and resilience of the human spirit. Through her unwavering belief in herself, perseverance, and dedication to self-care, she not only achieved her weight loss goals but also experienced profound personal growth. Sarah's story offers hope and encouragement to those embarking on their own journey towards a healthier and happier life, emphasizing the power of mindset, support, and perseverance in creating lasting positive change.

In conclusion, obesity is a significant public health concern that requires action from individuals, families, and communities. By working together to address the complex factors that contribute to obesity, we can reduce the burden of chronic diseases and improve the health and well-being of individuals and communities around the world.